I am a Food Addict, Now What?

Elisa R. Calleiro

Starting Point

If you received this workbook as a gift from a friend or loved one, trust me you are not alone. I too have been the recipient of many diet books. There are a whole group of us, receiving diet books from people that hope we can find lasting peace with food; however, **most food addicts <u>don't need</u> diet books**.

We are entrenched with dietary and caloric knowledge. We know what to do, and yet we can't seem to do it. This complexity led me to get real with myself. "Why don't I live healthy?"

"I know what is good for me, right?" - <u>*I answered "yes"*</u>   What is your answer: _____

"I don't always do it, why not?" - <u>*I don't really know*</u>   What is your answer: _____

My doctors and counselors had never peeled back this layer, so it became the basis of this workbook.

1. **Why do I not make time for my own health?**
2. **What do I make time for in my life?**

I started thinking, pouring over my journals, workout logs, and books.

"I start. I stop. I binge. I start. I stop. I binge. I try again. I binge. I cry. I almost give up." - What is this?

This is a cycle.

All around the world, daily battles are being repeated with a number of pawns replacing food. For some people the pawns are multiple partners, high risk activities, drugs, or excess work; for others it is food.

Are you like me? Are you a food addict? _____

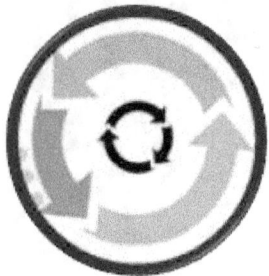

What dreams do you put on hold for food:

_____

_____

_____

I decided to write this workbook to help me stay on track after I noticed something about my life as a food addict. I know the methods of several diets and workouts.

In fact, I know more about becoming healthy than those who don't struggle with food. Food addicts are acutely aware of health, so why aren't we healthy?

What am I waiting for to become the healthiest version of myself?

_____

Basis of the Book

Why do I not make time for my own health?	What do I make time for in my life?

Come back to this page as you make new self-discoveries along the way. Fill in a few starting ideas now.

Check in (For those with Insurance)

Now is the time to form your check in list. It is time to make a clear assessment of where you are and who will help you. You need to gather a few supplies for this section. This page isn't set in stone; you may want to make copies of the blank page to return to later. It will need to change as you do.

Support Systems

1. Primary care doctor _____ office number:_____
   - Have I had a recent physical?
   - Do I have any serious underlying health issues?
   - Am I taking any medicines?
   - Do any of those medicines interfere with my health?
   - Do I need to make any changes to my current health coverage to support my health?

2. Obesity Specialist or Nutritionist _____ office number:_____
   - Do I need to find a specialist?
   - Have I had a recent talk about my current health?
   - When did I last weigh in?
   - Is the plan I am using benefiting my health?

3. Psychiatrist or Counselor _____ office number:_____
   - Have I ever talked with someone about my health?
   - Do I need to seek someone new?
   - Is my current provider benefiting my health?

4. Trainer or Gym Staff _____ office number:_____
   - Have I had a recent physical?
   - Am I healthy enough to work out on my own?
   - Do I need support?
   - Do I want to join a gym?
   - Do I want to work out with friends?
   - What programs are available in my community?

5. Support Group _____ Contact number, website, or email:_____
   - Is there community support for healthy living near me?
   - Is there anyone else who is dealing with this at work, school, or in my neighborhood?
   - Are there any meetings I would benefit from attending?
   - Do I need to consider inpatient treatment for eating disorders?

6. Close Friend _____ number:_____
   - Can I count on this person to understand my tough days?

Check in (For those without Insurance)

Now is the time to form your check in list. Don't panic if you don't have easy access to insurance or financial tools that other people do. You can still focus on your health. This page isn't set in stone; you may want to make copies of the blank page to return to later. It will need to change as you do.

Support Systems

1. A local doctor or health clinic _____ office number:_____
   - Have I had a recent physical?
   - Are there community locations offering free screenings?
   - Do I have any serious underlying health issues?
   - Do I need access to any medicines prescribed?
   - Does the doctor/clinic offer reduced cost, samples, coupons, or generic prescriptions?
   - Do any of my medicines interfere with my health?
   - Do I need to make any changes to my current health coverage to support my health?

2. Obesity Specialist /Nutritionist /Community Group_____ numbers:_____
   - Are there any free local meetings I can attend?
   - Have I had a recent talk about my current health?
   - Have I researched the papers and online?
   - When did I last weigh in?

3. Community Mental Health/ Counselor _____ office numbers:_____
   - Have I ever talked with someone about my health?
   - Do I need to talk with someone about eating disorders?
   - Are my current actions benefiting my health?
   - Are there any free community resources to help me?

4. Trainer/gym staff/local group _____ _____numbers:_____
   - Am I healthy enough to work out on my own?
   - Do I need support? Do I want to work out with friends?
   - What low cost or free programs are available in my community?

5. Support Group _____ Contact number, website, or email:_____
   - Have I found anything in my community that supports healthy thinking?
   - Is there anyone else who is dealing with this at work, school, or in my neighborhood?
   - Are there any free community support meetings that I would benefit from attending?
   - Have I found any online resources or support groups that are healthy?

6. Close Friend _____ number:_____
   - Can I count on this person to understand my tough days?

Now What?

If you sense that something isn't benefiting your health, you may be right. When it comes down to it, you may be asking more questions than when we started. The two main questions are still relevant.

By "checking in" you addressed part of the "**Why don't I make time for my own health?**" question. Now it's time to move on to the "**What do I make time for in my life?**" question.

_____

Let's start by charting a typical day:

After **waking up** I make time for..._____
_____

At **breakfast time** I make time for... _____
_____

Mid-morning I make time for..._____
_____

At **lunch time** I make time for..._____
_____

Mid-afternoon I make time for..._____
_____

At **dinner time** I make time for..._____
_____

Mid-evening I make time for..._____
_____

At **bedtime** I make time for..._____
_____

My **priorities** seem to be..._____

Thinking Patterns

For this activity you will need to circle the words which you feel a connection to in your life.

Smart	Funny	Diligent	Lazy	Tired	Faithful	Sad	Happy
Lonely	Hurt	Fed up	Sassy	Starved	Strong	Let down	Listless
Open	Benevolent	Quiet	Loud	Dynamic	Doubtful	Desire	Loved
Short	Gentle	Tall	Disorganized	Positive	Psycho	Weak	Sharing
Arrogant	Outgoing	Helper	Peppy	Teacher	Organized	Healthy	Huge
Mannered	Full	Distant	Serious	Rich	Alone	Hated	Poor

Do the words you feel connected to have more positive or negative connotations? _____

Did you choose any contradictory words? If you did, then what conflicting connections are there?

_____
_____
_____

What issues shape your everyday life or thinking patterns?

_____
_____
_____

What lifelong goals did you have as a child?

_____
_____
_____

Have your goals changed throughout the years?

_____
_____
_____

Is there anyone who you feel understands the real you?

_____
_____
_____

What does it take for people to understand the real you?

_____
_____
_____

Understand and Categorize Triggers

Check out my list on the left to brainstorm your own ideas.

3 Hidden Stress Thoughts
(Thoughts that keep me up at night...)

What if I never meet my goals?

I don't want to run into old friends

What if I never make peace with myself?

3 Hidden Stress Thoughts
(What thoughts keep you up at night?)

_____

_____

_____

Celebration/Life (Excuses)

It's a Birthday, back to normal soon.

It's Thanksgiving, back to normal soon.

It's Christmas, back to normal soon.

We're on a cruise, back to normal soon.

Celebration/Life (Excuses)

_____

_____

_____

_____

Coping with Work

Just one more project to go...

No time for a real lunch.

No more diet talk at the table.

Office potluck and snacks...

Coping with Work

_____

_____

_____

_____

Friends & Family

Let's eat out (lots of foods available)

Cooking for family (picky eaters)

Take out. I don't feel like cooking.

It tastes good, and I'm fitting in...

Friends & Family

_____

_____

_____

_____

Understand and Categorize Triggers (Continued)

Pain (Physical)

Heartburn doesn't seem better, ever

Migraines – make the pain go away

Joints and muscles ache (workout)

Pain (Emotional)

I will never be rid of stretch marks

Why is this weight my battle?

I don't get good attention, ever.

No one sees my real value now.

Coping with Unfairness

I was born with heart issues.

No one else in my family is overweight.

I want to be known for my life skills.

I'm doing this journey on my own

Surviving Crisis

Inappropriate attention

Finding a job in time of recession

Unplanned Pregnancy

Deaths in the family

Separation or Divorce

Deep anguish or heartache

Pain (Physical)

_____

_____

_____

Pain (Emotional)

_____

_____

_____

_____

Coping with Unfairness

_____

_____

_____

_____

Surviving Crisis

_____

_____

_____

_____

_____

_____

Identifying and Destroying Self-Hatred

When I was attending college there were several incidents which shaped my perspective. One incident which sticks out within my mind is the day when a guy didn't hold the door for me. It was raining, and I was carrying books. The guy didn't even seem to notice me. He opened the door immediately for the smaller girl behind me. It was a strange moment.

That same scene replayed itself again when I entered the workforce. I was lugging a huge load upstairs. A guy walked past, and he didn't even blink. That same guy helped many other petite women. He never noticed my need. I started to despise my own invisibility, and I believed it was a part of me. I noticed that I was often larger than my male co-workers and friends. I out-sized them, and I honestly felt as though I lost my femininity.

Do you feel like you have lost anything in your pursuit of food?

_____

_____

_____

I stopped buying clothes that fit my new plus size. I covered up in huge coats, sweaters, layers of ill-fitting clothes. I didn't worry about my hair. My twisted thought process: "Why fix the shingles when all the walls are falling down?" I literally thought of myself as an irreparable project.

Do you feel like food and weight has become uncontrollable in your life? What does that thought do to you?

_____

_____

_____

I saw my own life as mundane, and I started to experience other mental instabilities. My tendency to hoard papers, books, journals, boxes, photos, and knickknacks was exacerbated by my self-imposed isolation. I was punishing myself for being overweight, or not fitting into my old clothes. I could not accept that I still had value.

Do you punish yourself?

_____

_____

_____

I worked longer hours, watched more TV, and gravitated toward food. The cycle was unending. I felt sad because I was fat, so I ate. I felt sad that I over ate, so I punished myself. I felt bad because I was self-punishing, and my binging cycles continued.

Are there any self-destructive cycles in your own life?

_____

_____

_____

_____

Expose your Perceptions

What do you feel when you see <u>obese</u> people? Cut out 2 pictures and place them here. Write your thoughts and emotions about the images you find. Are you prejudiced in any way?

Image#1:

Image #2

What do you feel when you see anorexic people? Cut out 2 pictures and place them here. Write your thoughts and emotions about the images. Are you prejudiced in any way?

Image #1:

Image #2:

Write out any anxiety that surfaced in finding or decribing the extreme body type pictures.

What is <u>Body Image</u>?

Try to define the word "body" and the word "image"

_____
_____
_____
_____
_____
_____

How does the dictionary define "<u>healthy</u>"?

_____
_____
_____
_____
_____
_____

Do people of all shapes and sizes live healthy lives?

_____
_____
_____

Interview one person who you consider to be <u>unhealthy</u>, and try asking that person to define body image.

_____
_____
_____
_____

Interview one person who you consider to be <u>healthy</u>, and try asking that person to define body image.

_____
_____
_____
_____

Think of two things that <u>you are currently doing</u> that contribute to being healthy.

_____
_____
_____
_____

Think of two things that you <u>would be willing to try</u> to contribute to being healthy.

_____
_____
_____
_____
_____

What does my body say about me?

Draw an image which you see as representation of your own silhouette. It doesn't have to be pretty. Remember other people cannot chisel away the pounds to see the successful, smart person you are.

Until they invent a device to help us instantly see values, talents, and skills we will have to depend on our projected image.

It took me years to realize that people actually size me up in such simplistic ways.

I see my entire substance, and I assume people reject me on the sum total of who I am.

When I really am honest with myself, they have rejected a false version of me.

The body image I project says: "I don't care about fitness, health, or even putting my needs as a priority. I will do whatever the world needs me to do; because I don't make time to love myself."

Are you projecting the wrong image to the world around you?

_____

What do my needs look like?

If I take time to address my needs would I ever look so run down, pushed over, flabby, or exhausted. Sometimes I don't even put into words what I want or need. I assume that my needs will be met. When they aren't met, I assume that is life. I noticed that most healthy people verbalized needs frequently.

Have you ever verbalized what you really need?

_____
_____
_____

Are other people aware of your needs?

_____
_____
_____

Are there any needs which you are hesitant to say out loud for yourself?

_____
_____
_____

What needs are you currently meeting in your own life?

_____
_____
_____

Is there anything healthy that you really want for yourself?

_____
_____
_____

In what ways does food meet any of your wants or needs?

_____
_____
_____

In what ways does food replace your real wants or needs?

_____

Who are my true dependents?

This may not apply to every overeater or food addict, but it applies to me. I run out of time for myself and miss opportunities for my own self-improvement because I am trying to help capable people too much. I am trying to help everyone succeed, and yet I am not helping myself. I ignore my own needs too often. If a person is not truly my dependent (young or disabled), should I give them all of my time?

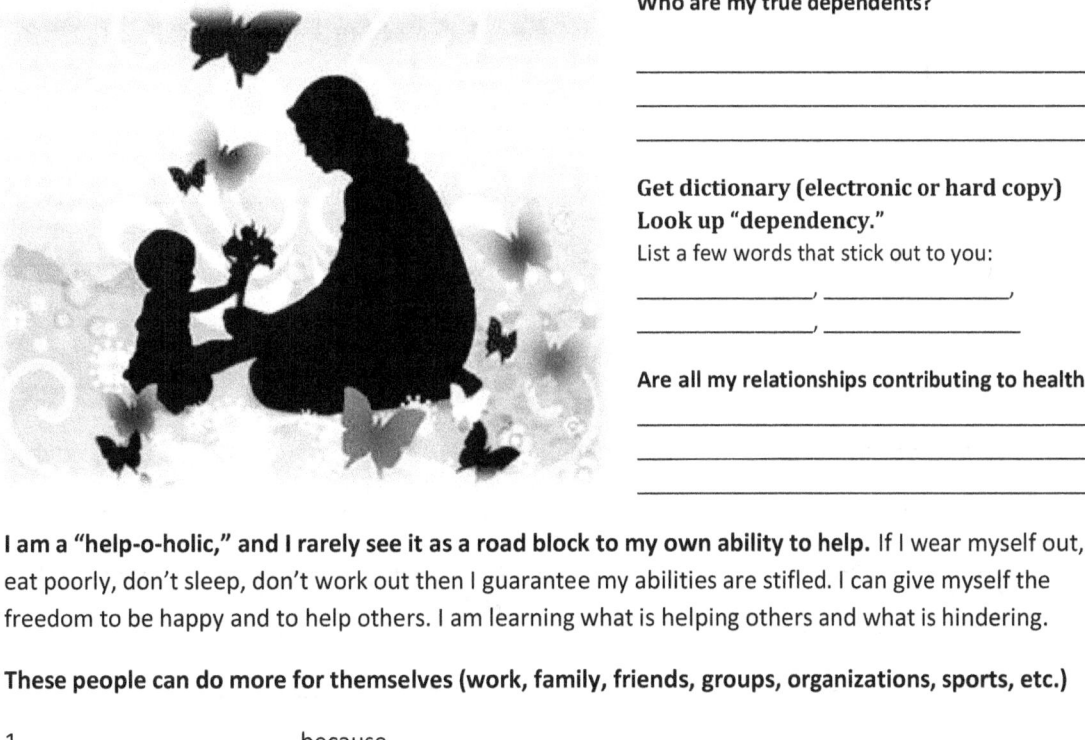

Who are my true dependents?

_____

_____

_____

Get dictionary (electronic or hard copy)
Look up "dependency."
List a few words that stick out to you:

_____, _____,

_____, _____

Are all my relationships contributing to health?

_____

_____

_____

I am a "help-o-holic," and I rarely see it as a road block to my own ability to help. If I wear myself out, eat poorly, don't sleep, don't work out then I guarantee my abilities are stifled. I can give myself the freedom to be happy and to help others. I am learning what is helping others and what is hindering.

These people can do more for themselves (work, family, friends, groups, organizations, sports, etc.)

1._____ because _____

2._____ because _____

3._____ because _____

4._____ because _____

5._____ because _____

Did you find any "hidden time" along your list of capable people depending on you? _____

I constantly return to the simplicity of a quote I found while attending college. It even applies to me.

"Never do for someone what they can do for themselves." -Saul Alinsky

Picture time

This page is one that may be very humbling and difficult to do in just one sitting. It took me a while to formulate exactly what hurts and losses I was experiencing on a daily basis due to my food addiction.

Pull out pictures that you have around the house or online. Recount the full toll of your addiction. Write words or emotions that you feel when looking through the images of you with friends or family.

Past Images

_____

_____

_____

_____

_____

_____

_____

_____

_____

_____

_____

_____

_____

_____

_____

_____

Present Images

_____

_____

_____

_____

_____

_____

_____

_____

_____

_____

_____

_____

_____

_____

_____

_____

Visualize the Victory

I wasn't always morbidly obese. I was a student athlete all through late elementary to mid-high school. I wasn't a small person, but I didn't always feel so bulky. I ate in excess at times, and even hid food as a child, but I wasn't drastically out of control. I was an isolated college student when food addiction took over my life.

When did you notice food becoming your main priority?

_____
_____
_____

My body does have a natural tendency to hold weight, and since I was young it never hid my caloric intake. In some ways I can be thankful for this. I won't have any hidden killer heart attack. I won't have any drop dead out of nowhere scenario. I have always had my health thrown in my face. Every visit to the doctor has felt horrible. I cannot remember a time when the scale didn't bring me shame. I have dealt with abnormal weight my whole life.

How long has weight been an issue in your life?

_____
_____
_____
_____

Fortunately there are a few other things which I have dealt with my whole life too. One of those things was running late. I finally worked on that this year; because, there is always time to re-learn. It felt odd to clock in before the required time. My other life-long struggle is hoarding. There are pictures of me as a child surrounded by items I couldn't sort through in my room. I can still hear my parents; "If you will finish cleaning your room you can…" there was always some incentive. It has been the same with my weight. "If you will only… then you can…"

What do you tell yourself that you can do when you conquer food or weight issues?

_____
_____
_____
_____

Over the past 2 years I have enjoyed not running late and not hoarding. It is new. I've taken over 16 trips to Goodwill. I still battle "the need for stuff" and the "minimalist lifestyle". I am not completely organized. There are places in my home which look like they belong to Monk, the OCD detective, and some that could be a ex-hoarder's new residence. I am a walking contradiction at times. It is a process, but I do see huge victories in these 2 areas.

Are you noticing any areas of victory in your own life?

_____
_____
_____
_____

Complex Individuals

There are trendy bumper stickers which say, "Take life a day at a time." I just want to ask them, "Is there any other way?" That catch phrase sounds so helpful, but in my own life it hasn't been. I have tried a lot of different solutions to food addiction. Solutions work for a while, but then I emerge. I am a complex person. We all are.

In what ways is your situation more complex than other people that you know?

_____

_____

_____

If there was an instant, non-complicated "fix" for weight loss, Oprah Winfrey would be beyond skinny. That woman is the smartest, most driven woman alive, and yet she struggles, like me, with food choices and genetics.

Once I realized food addiction was a much more complex issue than dieting, I finally found freedom. I will never win the war against "fat" and "thin." I will find sanity and make peace with a healthier version of myself. I will live a healthy lifestyle, and whatever comes out on the other side is who I am.

What realizations have you made along this journey so far?

_____

_____

_____

I found a couple of neat ways to visualize what might come out on the other side of a healthy lifestyle. Being healthy isn't impossible for me. I can't get my mind to wrap around the idea of being thinner. It hasn't stuck in years. I do however know how to become healthy. I need to work out and eat healthier. This shift in thinking has propelled me to the gym. It wasn't pretty, and my gym shorts didn't fit that nicely, but I went.

Have you done anything uncomfortable lately to reach for health?

_____

_____

_____

_____

When I began to dwell on health, I no longer dreaded the 110lb teenage girl who worked at the front desk. We are both unique. I let her help me weigh in. I told her about my weight and my heart issues. I felt "ok" with me. I was enough. I still didn't make much eye contact with the guys on staff. I'll leave that for the next visits.

What bothers you about getting healthy? Are there any barriers or frustrations which you anticipate?

_____

_____

_____

_____

Create, Draw, or Paste - "Healthy Life"

This is the space to collage your image of "Healthy People."
You can use images from magazines, your own drawings, or even photographs to illustrate.

This is the space to collage your image of "Healthy Hobbies."
You can use images from magazines, your own drawings, or even photographs to illustrate.

This is the space to collage your image of "Healthy Me."

Place an image of your face onto this page within a lifestyle of health. Envision your new life and body.

Feeling like an Outsider to Society

Sometimes I would watch television shows or see people and think, "How are they so fit?" There are so many places in which I feel like I cannot relate. I feel strange or unworthy of being a part of the group.

This feeling may only apply to a small group of weight loss candidates. I am a lifelong weight battler. I have a bulk of weight to lose. I am also a woman. I have been raised in certain cultures and surrounded by certain images or ideas. You may not relate to this section, or you may be thinking, "That's me too!"

Are there any places in which you have been feeling or acting like an outsider? Did you hold back today?

Mine – (Today) _I didn't go to any New Year's Eve parties tonight, like I wanted._

Yours- (Today)_____

Mine- (Recently) _I didn't post family photos from recent holiday celebrations_.

Yours- (Recently)_____

Mine- (In the Past) _I didn't go to a waterfall outing with friends in Costa Rica._

Yours- (In the Past) _____

Try writing a narrative about a moment you felt like an outsider. Get creative. (My stories would include: pools, the gym, mall stores, 5k races, fashion shows, cruises, the beach, clubs, or blind dates.)

_____
_____
_____
_____
_____
_____
_____
_____
_____
_____
_____
_____
_____
_____
_____
_____
_____
_____

Counting the Number of Attempts

This is a part when I am getting really honest with myself, and hopefully you can too. I have tried to quit being overweight so many times. I lose track of all the ways. Put a timer on a counter or your nightstand.

Set it for 3 minutes. (Take more time or pages if you need it. This is about seeing and learning patterns.)

Do your best to name all the <u>attempts</u> you have made to lose weight, <u>why it failed</u>, <u>how you felt</u>.

~~~~~~

Group Weight Loss   _didn't relate/commit to program - cheated, worked out but didn't count pts._

I like doing weight loss on my own. I don't like incentives. Felt unbalanced.

~~~~~~

1._____   _____

_____

2._____   _____

_____

3._____   _____

_____

4._____   _____

_____

5._____   _____

_____

6._____   _____

Almost Failures

No matter what mainstream media declares, we are all an important part of society. The uniqueness of each individual is remarkable. While we experience struggles and victories in different arenas, we are still connected in our humanity. There is probably not a person alive who has not experienced failure at some point. In fact, history is full of successful people who once failed miserably at things.

Try researching a few of the people from history who were not successful in their early attempts. There are many inventors, explorers, and scientists who almost never met their own goals. They could have retreated in dismay, but they persevered against all odds. We know their names today because they did.

For this section you may need access to a library or computer; list 5 people who were almost failures.

*Example: **Thomas Edison** experienced setbacks but finally succeeded in creating the light bulb.*

*This person's complex setbacks included: an incredible number of failures in work, school, and hobbies

1._____ experienced setbacks but finally succeeded in _____

*This person's complex setbacks included: _____

2._____ experienced setbacks but finally succeeded in _____

*This person's complex setbacks included: _____

3._____ experienced setbacks but finally succeeded in _____

*This person's complex setbacks included: _____

4._____ experienced setbacks but finally succeeded in _____

*This person's complex setbacks included: _____

5._____ experienced setbacks but finally succeeded in _____

*This person's complex setbacks included: _____

Do you see a trend; is there anything you have in common with these people? _____

_____

_____

_____

_____

The Daily Barrage

At some point, about a year ago, I started noticing the insane amount of daily visual and auditory messages regarding food. I once counted 39 separate food enticements on my daily path. Sometimes I take pictures of the most tempting advertisements, and other times I log them into a blog or journal.

For example: I am pumping gas at a gas station, and a visual poster of a "sticky doughnut" greets me at the side of the pump. I take note of it, pulling out my cell phone to take a quick picture. "Wow that one nearly got me, because I am actually hungry and didn't think to pack a snack." Binge averted; it is **level 2**.

Logging the visual assault to my "food sanity" helped me learn to be aware of my surroundings. Now that I am aware of this daily barrage, I started fighting it differently. I saw the marketing game going on all around me. The **level** that I wrote above came from my own ranking system. You may want one too.

Do you want to create a ranking system? Y or N

(Check out mine below for basic ideas and revamp it)

If it includes one of these elements it is a **level one**, two elements becomes **level two** and so on...

1. **Free/Fundraiser**– no cost or benefits others
2. **Fast Food** – simple, easy
3. **Filler** – I am hungry
4. **Fitting in** – everyone is doing it
5. **Food I love** – some level of emotional payoff

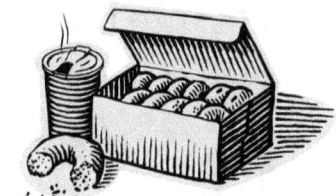

A **level 5** food encounter will be a hard one to forget. I will often fixate on this food even if I don't eat it at the time. I will think about it for a while and then go buy it secretly when I am on my own.

The newest **level 4** that I am battling has come at work. I saw a co-worker eating something that would set me on a spiral. A charity fundraiser packed with sugar goodies. This snack appeals to me on **4 levels**.

Does it always work? No, and I wish it was that easy. I now win 4 out of 5 battles, and I'm aiming higher.

What is your realistic goal? I will aim for winning _____ **out of** _____ food battles this week. Be honest.

Explain your thinking with your goal for this week. Why did you pick this goal number?

_____

_____

_____

A Food Threat Ranking System

To conquer my greatest food addiction threats I have a few strategies that typically work. I always have to keep changing things up as I become more aware of my thinking patterns. I now categorize threats. These are mine: Free/Fundraiser, Fast Food, Fitting in, Filler, and Food I love

Your top 5 food threats:

1._____ because _____

2._____ because _____

3._____ because _____

4._____ because _____

5._____ because _____

Most of my biggest food threats come from being unprepared. I made the mistake of waiting a really long time to eat the other day, and I set myself up for failure. Believe it or not there was a man selling donuts door to door as a fundraiser for his national track team. I was almost caught in this food trap.

This threat included: **Food I love**, **Fast Food**, **Fundraiser**, and **Filler**

Thankfully my healthy friend suggested that we give a monetary donation and not take any doughnuts.

_____

For this next part you will need to evaluate your daily path:

Does my drive home pass any major food threats?

Does my work environment have any major food threats?

Does my home hold any major food threats?

Do my relatives or close friends' homes present any major food threats?

Do I purposefully take or avoid different routes based on my addiction?

Do I plan ahead with how to deal with food threats?

_____

I noticed something else about this healthy friend of mine. She always carries healthy snacks.

Do you have healthy snacks on hand at all times? _____

Try, Try, Try – Slip

There are many great addiction websites that helped me to put my mind around why quitting anything is tough. According to some websites I visited for research about addiction, slip ups and give ups are a part of the quitting process. There is a great saying among the addiction community.

"Just don't do it, ever"

"Not ever?" I try to bargain. What panic filled thoughts fill your mind when you read this quote?

_____

I took this quote to mean not binging or making excuses, because <u>not eating</u> is <u>not an option</u>.

I must not allow food to rule my thinking. If I want to try something delicious, then I will allow myself to try it without binging on the entire box or bag. I can regulate my intake, and if I cannot regulate myself with certain foods then I will eliminate these binge trigger foods from my household purchases.

For example: If I can't avoid buying binge items at the gas station then I will take steps to avoid going inside (paying at pump.) If I can't avoid buying binge items at the grocery store then I will seek help.

This chart is what happens in my own life every time I try to conquer my food addiction. You can discuss specific addiction studies with a counselor or doctor. They have un-ending resources at their fingertips.

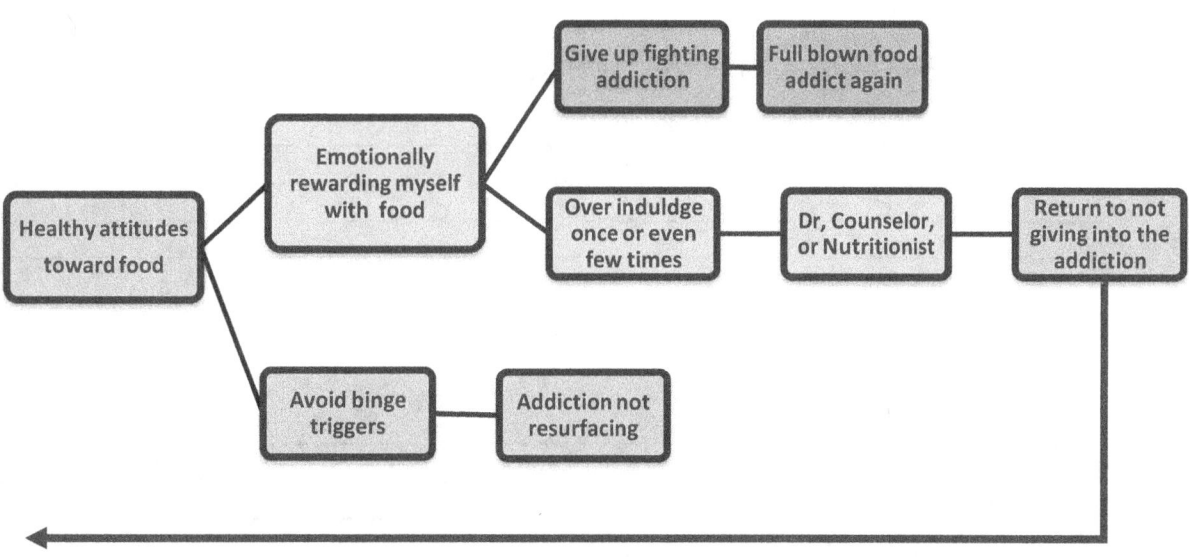

The Taste of Success

There is something so rewarding about the tastes of certain foods. In fact there are even foods which are being engineered to activate our reward sensations. Foods which are high in fat often taste great.

Identify some of your favorite crave foods which you know are high in fat or calories:

1.	2.	3.	4.
5.	6.	7.	8.
9.	10.	11.	12.
13.	14.	15.	16.

When you encounter these foods what concepts, images, or sensations come into your mind?

_____
_____
_____

In what ways are these foods controlling your thinking?

_____
_____
_____

Are you willing to have limited interactions with these foods?

_____
_____
_____
_____

Are you willing to replace any of these foods?

_____
_____
_____
_____

"Are you ready to order?"

Today I faced one of my most frustrating items as a food addict: **"The Restaurant Menu"**

I read and re-read the menu several times to find anything that appealed to my **picky tastes**, to my **tight budget**, and to my **pursuit of health**.

There were not <u>any</u> items which seemed to hold all of these things.

Daily Specials:

½ Order of Delayed Guilt - $18

Extra Large Workout - $26

10 Sizes from My Goals - $15

A Side of Avoiding - $11

Frustrated Aspirations - $34

The organization of a menu is often the main source of irritation for me. I will give up looking for healthy items if I cannot follow the layout.

Taking time to know what I want is crucial to my new healthy decisions.

Something I am trying now is to stop ordering with only my favorite tastes in mind. I have to allow myself to feel a bit of anxiety.

I take note of the anxiety level.

I pause and find a way to deal with food as fuel, not pleasure.

I try to think about non-edible pleasures (fun hobbies) as I order.

I only feel weak when I don't anticipate the anxiety that will be present in food-centered activities.

I feel strong when I prepare myself for upcoming stressors.

There isn't a perfect way to deal with restaurant menus, but there is a healthy way to approach them.

Finding Peace with Food:

Better Eye Sight - $12

No Heavy Feeling - $23

Running on the Beach - $17

A Good Attitude - $10

Immune Boost- $29

The Role of Food

I am scared that if I don't have food as pleasure anymore my life will just be:

_____

_____

_____

Food means _____ to me. It is my _____

Everyone around me seems to view food as_____

Healthy people find pleasure in_____

One healthy thing that I have always dreamed of trying is:

_____

_____

_____

Interview 3 people about the role that food plays in their life:

1. (Unhealthy)_____
   _____
   _____

2. (Moderately Healthy)_____
   _____
   _____

3. (Very Healthy) _____
   _____
   _____

Life-Long Changes

As I started to apply the things I've learned through writing this workbook, I noticed setbacks. I resist change, and I fall apart when the changes are too drastic, too broad, or too unstable.

These aspects of change applied to my individual journey:

1. **I must make changes slowly and methodically**

Changing from unhealthy eating to drastic calorie restriction and lifestyle overhaul didn't last. What does seem to work for me is stepping down, item by item. I replace one unhealthy food or habit each week, and for some reason this seems to help me stick with the changes. I had to fix my breakfast habits before moving on to fixing lunch and dinner. I worked with breakfast until I figured out a few healthy items that I do like to eat. I started with some moderately healthy items and am now moving on to even healthier choices. It took about a year to accomplish this process matching my likes with healthy items.

2. **I must make changes based on my individual circumstances**

I had to be honest with myself and with my health providers about my specific set of health complications. I have had to change medicines, counselors, jobs, and my hobbies to find health.

3. **I must think healthy to be healthy**

I feel like it is impossible to obtain true physical health without balancing emotional and mental health. I have had the most success with my pursuit of health when I am honest with myself and my doctors.

Attitudes toward change: (Circle one or more of the options and then evaluate your thinking patterns)

1. Change for me (**takes a long time**) or (**happens suddenly**)
2. I am (**comfortable**) or (**uncomfortable**) making lots of changes
3. I can change (**1**), (**2**), or (**3**) meals from unhealthy to healthy at a time
4. People say that I am (**set in my ways**) or (**changing my ways frequently**)
5. I find new things (**great**), (**scary**), (**interesting**), (**confusing**), (**frustrating**), (**odd**), (**ok**)
6. All around me the world is (**staying the same**) or (**changing**)
7. I am a huge fan of (**change**), (**habits**), (**routine**)
8. There are never enough hours in the day for (**trying new things**) or (**my traditional hobbies**)
9. If I could travel anywhere I would (**visit somewhere new**) or (**return to place I liked before**)
10. Words that best describe change include: (**overwhelming**), (**new**), (**fun**), (**hard**), (**bothersome**)
11. In general the (**anxiety**) or (**fun**) of change contributes to my overall health
12. When people make changes, other people initially (**accept**) (**reject**) (**support**) these changes
13. The ideas that my friends or family have about change are (**healthy**) or (**unhealthy**)
14. Health (**is**) or (**is not**) worth making changes
15. (**Beginning**), (**Continuing**), (**Establishing**), (**Determining**) changes is crucial to life-long change

10 things I learned about my health

I have gained and lost massive amounts of weight multiple times, and I finally learned a few things.

1. A lot of diets are designed for people who are <u>not</u> seeking to be healthy.
2. Calories in many fad diets are restricted to half of what I actually need.
3. I'm not going to need to restrict my calories as low when my weight is high.
4. Nutritionists are not the enemy. A few specific tools and corrections go a long way.
5. I will try healthy research based methods, and I will ignore unrealistic or unhealthy fad diets.
6. Some people are healthy because they work hard, and some people are genetically advantaged.
7. If I am not genetically advantaged, then I will have to work hard.
8. If I mess up when trying to control my intake of calories, then I try again next meal. No big deal.
9. If I only focus on my food failures then I am guaranteed to repeat them.
10. I cannot expect just one diet or workout program to work. I will combine the best attributes.

_____

What concepts of health have given you the most setbacks? _____

What concepts of health have come easily to you? _____

Is there a person in your life who you consider to be a source of reliable health information? _____

Is there a place in which you feel most healthy? _____

_____

Try listing at least 10 things you recently learned about your health:

1. _____
2. _____
3. _____
4. _____
5. _____
6. _____
7. _____
8. _____
9. _____
10. _____

Overcoming Gym Shock

I chose a low maintenance plan for working out. When swimming took too much prep effort, I switched to jogging. When it got cold outside I joined a gym. I adapt with my body and my head. If you hate doing a type of activity then you will avoid it. It only makes sense. You have to like it.

If the gym is 30 miles out of your way, then it might be a pain to drive to every day. If you find something that naturally fits into your routine then it has a better chance of sticking.

Brainstorm ideas:

_____
_____
_____

Because I was so out of shape, I started every workout on an elliptical. I did what I could do. Before I started, a trainer suggested 5th level for 45 minutes. I nearly gasped.

There were a half a dozen buttons beeping at me, and there was the prompt to input my weight about 5 times throughout the workout. When I put my heavy weight for everyone to see, my calories ticked by so much quicker. Honestly, this visit was the first time I ever felt confident.

Is there one time in which you felt confident in your own skin?

_____
_____
_____

It was liberating to no longer fear my actual real weight. I tried the bikes after that. If I felt the bike was boring or too easy I switched back to the elliptical. After I felt really tired, I pushed a bit farther, then I quit for the day. I did the same thing, until I finally felt like trying something else.

What fears do you have about the gym or independent workouts?

_____
_____
_____

Group classes, weight lifting, yoga, everything ambitious can wait until the gym shock wears off. If I push too hard at the beginning then I quit faster. I push just hard enough and then I rest.

I pick back up at the gym the next day, or sometimes I just work out at home. I keep it simple. The finish line is reachable as long as I am still moving.

What if I miss a workout week/month?

As I discovered my passion for swimming, decent like for jogging, and tolerable attitude for aerobics; I had a few setbacks. There are always going to be setbacks to a great workout plan. I learned the major setbacks that I experience are not all that uncommon. You may encounter setbacks as well, so it is important to discuss them. I like to chart them to realize what I have overcome. I'm tougher than I look.

Sick days

These are spaces to list sick days

They are bound to happen, it's ok

Take time to recover then start back

Sick days (list dates)

_____

_____

_____

Family or Friend Crisis

We've all had crisis moments

That cannot wait, because

Someone needs us & life happens.

Document it here and start back.

Family or Friend Crisis

_____

_____

_____

_____

Injury/Surgery

I just heard a man talk about

This setback and I realized it is

So universal to have physical

Limitations from time to time

Follow doctors orders then start back

Injury/Surgery (list dates)

_____

_____

_____

_____

_____

Financial or Emotional Crisis

The economy dropped a lot of us

Into a spin we didn't see coming

Panic makes it hard to workout

Find your bearings and start back

Financial or Emotional Crisis

_____

_____

_____

_____

It's just a pound...activities

In the Gym

I try picking up free-weight while in the gym. If you don't know what free weight is, it is a non-attached weight. The machines are one form of weights, and the ones without the machines are free-weight (i.e. dumbbells, hand weights).

I feel how much the weight slows my arm. If I lose even 5 pounds, then I am no longer carrying that amount of weight. I vary the amount of weights that I lift based on my current goals.

To copy my methods try:
- ☐ 5 pounds*
- ☐ 10 pounds*
- ☐ 15+ pounds*

*Use personal safety and precautions with free-weight lifting. Please ask for assistance from gym staff. Avoid conditions of dropping the weight.

In the Grocery Store

Every time I need a perspective of just how much weight I carry every day, I try lifting a heavy 30 lb bag of dog food. I would need to carry 3 at a time to estimate the feeling of my 90lb excess.

To visualize a smaller loss I find a pound of sugar. If I fill up a shopping cart with even a few of the bags, then I start to get excited about the small improvements. If I need to lose 100lbs – I carry the weight of 100 bags of sugar. That is way too much to carry. My cart would be so full.

Here are a few household items that I like to use to visualize my weight loss goals.

These items weigh about 1lb	What items did you find?
Apples (3 medium)	_____
Bananas (3 medium)	_____
Bag of Sugar	_____
8 eggs with shells	_____
12 to 16 slices of bread	_____
2 cups or 4 sticks of Butter	_____
About 4 cups shredded cheese	_____

According to www.caloriesperhour.com: A pound of body fat equates to approximately 3500 calories. So if you have a calorie deficit of 500 calories, meaning that you burn 500 calories more than you eat each day, you would lose approximately one pound per week.

500 calories x 7 days in a week = 3500 calorie deficit* (1 pound weight loss)
*to know your specific basal metabolic rate (the number of calories per day your body burns) check with nutritionist or doctor

Getting specific is everything

Basal metabolic rate (the number of calories per day your body burns) is different for every person. It is based on age, gender, activity level, and current weight. Research yours with a nutritionist or doctor.

It is the main factor in the health equation. **Even if you work out every day, there will be no changes until you flip the deficit ratios.** You must know the basics of what your body needs to live healthy.

For example: My basic calories needed to function based on my age, gender, activity level, and current weight is 2373. If I eat that amount my body will remain the same weight.

If I reduce that by 500 calories a day, to lose a pound a week, my calorie goal for the day is 1873.

 I can then use my entire calorie counting tools to figure out meals and workouts.

I tend to check several sources and don't just go with the most optimistic. When I had trouble with budgets I used an envelope system to track spending amounts. I saw this method help me fiscally.

I can put the 1873 calories into chunks. I can laminate the amounts. As I "spend" the calories I can add them to the spent envelope. If I feel like I've gone over, then I can add that to a sheet (workout tally).

Any excessive calorie expenditures will break my calorie budget. This is the mindset I like to take.

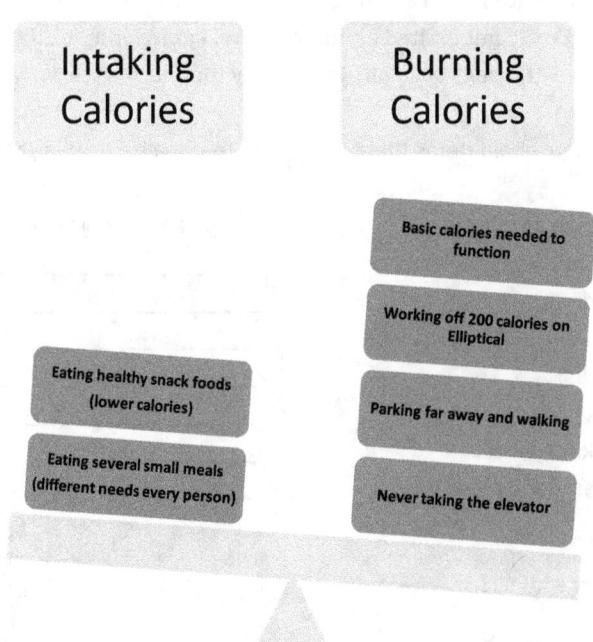

Lies to Justify my Binges

I generally have an intense awareness of what is good for me. I have illogical reasons and poor habits which get me off track. There are still many, many days when I listen to my physical hunger or "I deserve this..." thinking. I am working to illuminate my irrational thinking patterns, and I am contradicting them.

Lies I tell myself to justify my addiction:

I earned this

It's just a little bit

I will never reach my goal

It tastes so good, it can't be bad

I am tired of trying

I am never going to do this right

I am not going to stick with it

I was born like this

I am really hungry

People shouldn't judge me

I have hurts that no one understands

This is the last time I do this

I will not lose control

My situation is hopeless

People don't change

I can't change

Consistency is boring

I will deal with this tomorrow

Just one time

Lies I tell myself to justify my addiction:

_____

_____

_____

_____

_____

_____

_____

_____

_____

_____

_____

_____

_____

_____

_____

_____

_____

_____

_____

What is that Feeling?

Our bodies give us feedback. I have noticed that I often misread the cues. I mistake the cues for thirst, nausea, heartburn, heart ache, and loneliness as hunger. I am not very good at interpreting my body's signals or limits. **It has taken me years to realize that I often stuff food into the void of other things.**

What does true hunger feel like:_____

What does physical pain feel like:_____

What does heart ache feel like:_____

What does loneliness feel like:_____

What does frustration feel like:_____

Are there times when food is the only solution that comes to mind?_____

What is the solution for true hunger:_____

What is the solution for physical pain:_____

What is the solution for heart ache:_____

What is the solution for loneliness:_____

What is the solution for frustration:_____

How limited is food in solving true hunger:_____

How limited is food in solving physical pain:_____

How limited is food in solving heart ache:_____

How limited is food in solving loneliness:_____

How limited is food in solving frustration:_____

Who or What solves most of your problems:_____
Do you need to consider an inpatient setting for food addiction? Asking for additional help is healthy.

Workout Bag

I have a routine now that helps me with the "I don't feel like a workout" feeling. It is starting to help.

The **first step** is shopping for a few basic comfortable shorts, socks, shoes, and shirts.
The **second step** is keeping them clean. I have to frequently do laundry and put them all in one spot.
The **third step** is repacking the bag with adequate supplies.
The **fourth step** is putting on the workout clothes even when I don't feel like it. It adds motivation.

My List includes:

T-Shirt

Shorts/Pants

Undergarments & Socks

*Mp3 player (charged & loaded with music I like)

*Shoes

*Asthma Medicines

(*Stays in bag, everything else has to be repacked daily)

Your List includes:

_____

_____

_____

_____

_____

_____

This workbook is a brief overview of the complex systems at play in my lifelong health battles. As you finish reading, know that I am working and re-working every part in this workbook with you.

I still frustrate my doctors and nutritionists with my ups and downs with weight. This workbook is the culminating project of many months of working with them to find some solid ground to stand.

As I wrote this workbook for myself, I noticed many ways in which I still continue to struggle daily. I am motivated to keep trying, despite all odds, due to the inspiration of others. My life is changing.

The thing I most look forward to is a second edition to this workbook which includes your story, or perhaps reading the success story you begin writing today. I welcome all beneficial feedback.

- Elisa (ercalleiro@live.com)

Referenced Materials

Berridge KC, Robinson TE. What is the role of dopamine in reward: hedonic impact, reward learning, or incentive salience? Brain Res Rev. 1998;28:309-69.

Corwin RL, Grigson PS. Symposium overview. Food addiction: fact or fiction? J Nutr. 2009;139:617-9.

Davis C, Carter JC. Compulsive overeating as an addiction disorder. A review of theory and evidence. Appetite 2009;53:1-8.

Davis C, Strachan S, Berkson M. Sensitivity to reward: implications for overeating and overweight. Appetite 2004;42:131-8.

Gendall KA, Joyce PR. Characteristics of food cravers who binge eat. In: Hetherington MM, editor. Food cravings and addiction. Surrey (UK): Leatherhead Publishing; 2001. p. 567-84.

Kessler D. *The end of overeating: taking control of the insatiable North American appetite.* Toronto (ON): McClelland and Stewart; 2009.

Pelchat ML, Johnson A, Chan R, Valdez J, Ragland JD. Images of desire: food craving activation during fMRI. Neuroimage. 2004;23:1486-93.

Pelchat ML. Food addiction in humans. J Nutr 2009;139:620-2.

Additional resource sites:

- Mayo Clinic
  www.mayoclinic.com

- American Heart Association (AHA)
  1-800-242-8721 (1-800-AHA-USA-1)
  www.americanheart.org

- Centers for Disease Control and Prevention (CDC)
  www.cdc.gov

- American Cancer Society (ACS)
  1-800-227-2345 (1-800-ACS-2345)
  www.cancer.org

- U.S. Department of Health and Human Services
  http://www.hrsa.gov/

www.ingramcontent.com/pod-product-compliance
Lightning Source LLC
Chambersburg PA
CBHW081538280526
45788CB00010B/3278